BULLETPROOF
YOUR HAMSTRINGS

Optimizing Hamstring Function to End Pain and Resist Injury

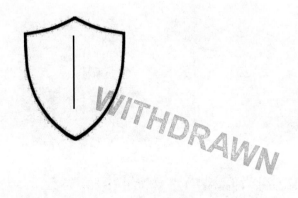

by

Jim Johnson, PT

Drawings by Eunice Johnson
Copyright © 2016 Jim Johnson
All Rights Reserved

This edition published by
Dog Ear Publishing
4010 W. 86th Street, Ste H
Indianapolis, IN 46268

www.dogearpublishing.net

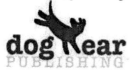

ISBN: 978-160844-562-2
Library of Congress Control Number: Applied For
This book is printed on acid-free paper.

Printed in the United States of America

I have given my best effort to ensure that this book is entirely based upon scientific evidence and not on intuition, single case reports, opinions of authorities, anecdotal evidence, or unsystematic clinical observations. Where I do state my opinion in this book, it is directly stated as such.

—*Jim Johnson, P.T.*

WWW.BODYMENDING.COM

TABLE OF CONTENTS

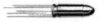

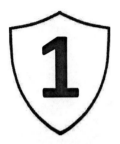

HOW TO BULLETPROOF YOUR HAMSTRINGS

Having "bulletproof" hamstrings is just a fun way of saying that you have hamstrings that are *pain-free* and *resistant to injury*. And if you look around, it probably won't take you long to find someone who has a hamstring problem. Each year, many active people experience one, and for many, it can become a nagging problem that never completely goes away. So just how does one go about "bulletproofing" their hamstrings from pain and injury?

Bulletproofing From Pain

Tackling hamstring pain is not hard if you go at it with the right approach. With the exception of new hamstring tears, when someone with a painful hamstring comes to see me, I keep one thought in the back of my mind – the pain is most likely the result of something not functioning properly. My job as a physical therapist, then, is not necessarily to come up with the precise cause of someone's pain, *which can often times be either elusive or controversial*, but rather to figure out what the hamstring muscle *isn't* doing that it normally should do. Using this approach during my evaluation, I routinely test the various functions of the hamstring muscle – such as how strong or flexible it is – so I can then determine what is or is not working up to par. Then, once the improper function has been identified, I can then choose a treatment that will restore it.

Consider the following list of possible treatments for a hamstring problem...

- injections

- heat

- stretching

- trigger point therapy

- pain medicines

- electrical stimulation

- mind-body techniques

- ice-packs

- massage

- strengthening exercises

- whirlpool

- surgery

As you can see from this rather lengthy list, medicine has come up with quite a wide range of treatment options when it comes to solving hamstring pain – and I'm sure there will be many more to come as time goes on.

While at first glance some of them appear to be *very* different from others, they all have a common thread running through them – *each of them is designed to restore or enhance the functioning of the hamstrings.*

Take a minute and think about it. Ice can reduce the swelling in your hamstring muscles so you can contract them easier. Pain medicine blocks the pain so they can be used without hurting. The most radical treatment of all, surgery, improves the function of the hamstring muscles by reattaching any torn ends so the hamstrings can create more force.

Thinking about treating hamstring pain in this manner can be quite useful when one is trying to figure out what to do about it. As an example, if the hamstring muscles are unable to stretch as far as they should, then a treatment is needed that will improve the hamstring's range of motion. And if the hamstring muscles are found to be weak, then a strengthening exercise would be in order. These, then, are the underlying principles this book will use to effectively eliminate any existing hamstring pain you might have once and for all...

> Most hamstring pain is the result of dysfunction. Restore the function with the proper treatment, and the pain will be relieved.

Bulletproofing from Injury

As we talked about earlier, having bulletproof hamstrings means having hamstring muscles that are pain-free and resistant to injury. Getting pain-free is a matter of treating anything that is not functioning properly and getting it up to par. So what's the plan for becoming resistant to injury?

Well, injury many times involves getting into a situation by chance. One example is falling down. Sometimes we just slip or trip – and the hamstrings get strained. Other examples are accidents that happen while lifting weights or playing a sport.

It's here that there's some good news and some bad news. The bad news is that there's not much you can do about chance occurrences or accidents most of the time – short of just "being careful". The good news, however, is that there is something you can do to eliminate, or at the very least *minimize* your chances of getting hurt when such unlucky events do occur – make sure your hamstrings are *optimally functioning*.

That's right, we're back to the idea of improving hamstring function once again. Just as improving hamstring function can get rid of pain, it can most certainly build hamstrings that are quite resistant to injury. In other words, hamstring muscles that have these four abilities can take a lot of abuse…

✓ **A Rock-Solid Base of Support**

✓ **Beefed-Up Concentric and Eccentric Strength**

✓ **An Optimal Strength Curve**

✓ **Maximal Flexibility**

The remainder of this book will go into great detail as to how you can quite easily develop each of the four abilities listed above that are absolutely essential to get 100% optimally functioning hamstring muscles, or in other words, *bulletproof* hamstrings. On the next page is a diagram that summarizes the concepts in this chapter that will be used in the pages that follow…

Normally functioning, pain-free hamstring muscles possesses four abilities:

- ✓ rock-solid base of support
- ✓ beefed-up concentric and eccentric strength
- ✓ an optimal strength curve
- ✓ maximal flexibility

Trauma, accidents, and aging changes

Loss of Function

Hamstrings lose one or more of the four abilities:

- ✓ rock-solid base of support
- ✓ beefed-up concentric and eccentric strength
- ✓ an optimal strength curve
- ✓ maximal flexibility

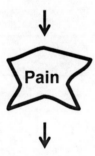

Pain

Regain lost function by doing specific exercises to restore the four abilities

***Bulletproof* Hamstrings**
Pain-free – Resistant to Injury

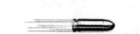

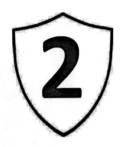

STEP ONE: STABILIZE YOUR PELVIS

Stabilize your pelvis. So what exactly does *that* mean? Well, first let's start with what a pelvis is, and then I'll tell you what it has to do with your hamstrings...

The Pelvis

Here's a basic picture of a human skeleton to get an overall view of things. The funny looking part in the middle of your body is your *pelvis...*

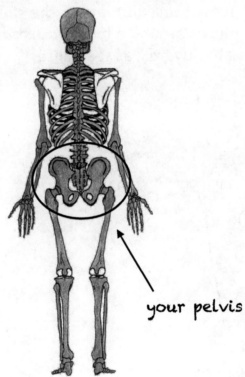

your pelvis

Figure 1. The pelvis - as it sits in the middle of your skeleton.

So that's what the pelvis looks like from *the front*. From the side, as it sits in your body, it looks something like this...

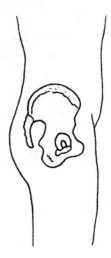

Figure 2. Side view of the pelvis.

But the pelvis doesn't just sit there in the same exact position all day long – it actually moves around a bit. For instance, the pelvis can rotate forward, as well as backwards, as seen here...

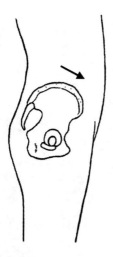

Figure 3. Side view of the pelvis rotating *forward*. Note how the low back curves in when this happens.

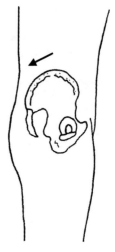

Figure 4. Side view of the pelvis rotating *backwards*. Note how the low back flattens out.

So what's all this got to do with your hamstrings? The answer lies in the fact that your hamstring muscles actually attach to your bony pelvis. Take a look...

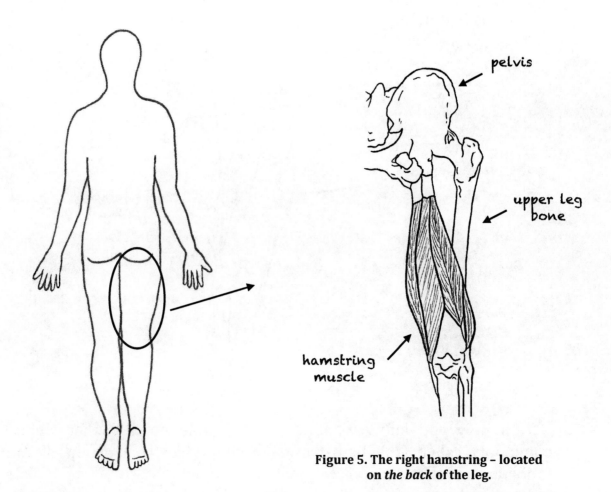

Figure 5. The right hamstring – located on *the back* of the leg.

Notice that the top ends of the hamstring muscle attach themselves to the pelvis – and the bottom ends to various points on your leg bones. Connecting in this manner, the hamstring muscle can do two main things - bend your knee (knee flexion), as well as help you bring your knee behind your body (extend your hip). As the picture shows, it's not just one big mass of muscle, but is actually made up of several distinct parts. On the next page are their names...

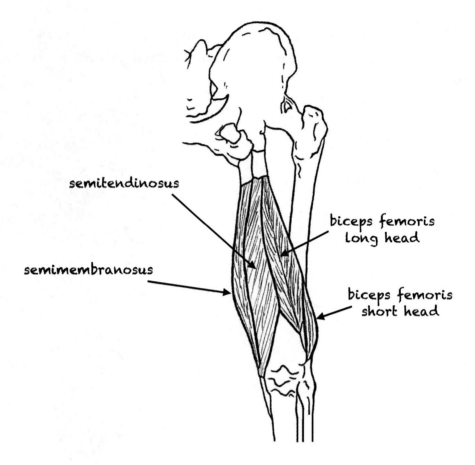

semitendinosus

biceps femoris
long head

semimembranosus

biceps femoris
short head

**Figure 6. The names of the individual muscles
that make up your hamstrings**

And now you know what a lot of people don't – that what is commonly called "the hamstring muscle" *is really* a group of **four** individual muscles!

So putting the information from the last few pages together, you can begin to see what the title of this chapter, "Stabilize Your Pelvis" has to do with bulletproofing your hamstrings. Since the hamstring attaches to the pelvis, and the pelvis moves, it is *very* important to make sure that you have good control of the pelvis – because excessive or uncontrolled motion of the pelvis *could* affect the well being and functioning of your hamstring muscles. On the next page is an example demonstrating how movement of the pelvis directly affects the hamstrings.

Standing still – pelvis is in a
middle or "neutral" position...

...but when you bend over – the pelvis
now rotates forward, which stretches
the hamstrings and makes it longer.

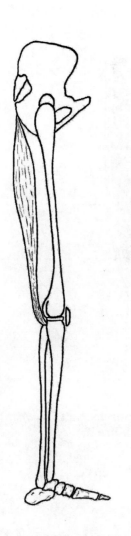

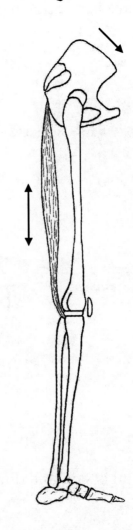

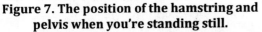

**Figure 7. The position of the hamstring and
pelvis when you're standing still.**

**Figure 8. The change in position of the pelvis
and hamstring *when you lean forward*.**

So this is how the motion of your pelvis – which moves around as you
do – can directly affect your hamstring muscle. The main point? Having
good control of your pelvis can definitely help bulletproof the
hamstrings that attach to it! And how do we control the pelvis?

Simply by strengthening the muscles that attach to the pelvis. Some might call them "the core" muscles – but since many people argue over which muscles actually make up "the core" – let's just call them "the trunk muscles." Here's a basic picture to show you where the trunk muscles are in relation to the pelvis...

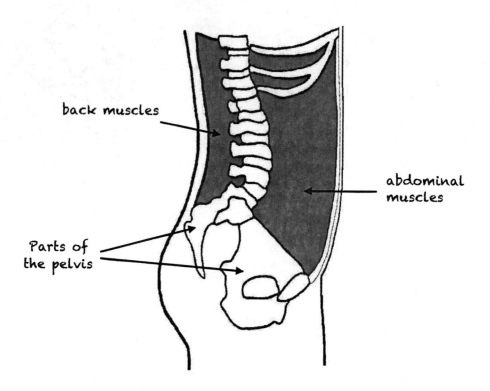

back muscles

abdominal muscles

Parts of the pelvis

Figure 9. The location of the trunk muscles that attach to the pelvis and help stabilize it.

So when all is said and done, it breaks down like this...

your pelvis moves

↓

your hamstring muscle is connected to your pelvis

↓

therefore, uncontrolled or excessive motion of the pelvis could affect the functioning of the hamstring muscle

↓

get better pelvic control by strengthening the trunk muscles

↓

bulletproof hamstrings

Pretty nifty, huh? Stabilizing the pelvis by strengthening the trunk muscles is probably one of the most overlooked treatments out there when it comes to hamstring problems. Take a look at this study I read one time that shows how exercising the trunk muscles can definitely affect the hamstring muscle...

- researchers took 30 volunteers with tight hamstrings and randomized them to one of two groups (Kuszewski 2009)
- one group did trunk stabilization exercises for 4 weeks
- the control group did nothing for 4 weeks
- both groups had the flexibility of their hamstrings measured before and after the 4-week study period
- at the end of the study, the group that did the trunk stabilization exercises actually increased the flexibility of their hamstring muscles, while the control group lost range of motion

Perhaps the most interesting thing here is that the hamstring muscles became more flexible, not by doing stretching exercises, but by doing *trunk stabilization* exercises. One can't say for sure, but it could be that the hamstring muscles get stiff trying to compensate for a lack of pelvic stability caused from weak trunk muscles. I definitely would like to see more research in this area!

And trunk stabilization exercises have also been shown in randomized, controlled trials to be effective in helping to treat hamstring *injuries* as well. Here's one such example...

- 24 athletes with an acute hamstring strain were randomized to one of two groups (Sherry 2004)
- the first group did icing, stretching, and hamstring strengthening exercises
- the second group did icing and agility and trunk stabilization exercises
- at the end of the study, the average time required to return to sports was 37 days in the first group, and 22 days in the trunk stabilization group

Apparently doing trunk stabilization exercises can help athletes with injured hamstrings get back into action sooner too! On the next page you'll find several trunk stabilization exercises – you only need to do *one*...

Trunk Muscle Strengthening Exercise
~The Plank~

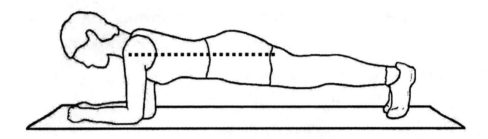

How to do it

This exercise is done quite easily. First, find a firm surface (the floor), get into the above position, and hold it there. How long? Work up to one full minute. When you can strictly hold the position in the picture for one full minute, make the exercise harder by wearing a backpack with a book or two in it - and begin working up to one full minute again.

- ✓ do one time a day, twice a week, separated by at least a day of rest in between sessions (i.e. Monday-Friday or Tuesday-Saturday)
- ✓ as you can see from the picture, only your elbows and toes should be touching the floor
- ✓ it is VERY important to try and keep your trunk straight as the dotted line shows – the exercise is over when you are unable to keep your trunk straight any longer
- ✓ use a towel or pillow under you elbows for comfort if needed

---

It's a Fact!
The following published EMG studies have confirmed that your front and back trunk muscles are coactivated when doing this specific exercise.

✓ **Snarr 2014, Comfort 2011**

Alternate Trunk Muscle Strengthening Exercise
~The Bird Dog~

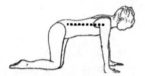

Starting Position

1. You should be on all fours.
2. Your trunk should be straight as the dotted line shows.

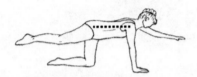

Exercise Movement

1. Raise the right leg and left arm up, close to the horizontal, *at the same time*.

2. Hold for a second, then lower them both.

3. Keep your trunk straight, as the dotted line shows, while doing the exercise.

4. Repeat, except this time, raise the left leg and the right arm up, close to the horizontal, at the same time.

5. Hold for a second, then lower, trying to keep the trunk straight.

6. Do this over and over again, *alternating* the right leg/left arm with the left leg/right arm - eventually working up to a total of 20 times (that would be a total of 20 with the right leg/left arm and 20 with the left leg/right arm).

7. When you can do this exercise 20 times in a row (a total of 20 times with the right leg/left arm and 20 times with the left leg/right arm) with the trunk straight, add a 1 or 2-pound ankle weight and begin working your way up to 20 times again.

8. Do one time a day, twice a week, separated by at least a day of rest in between sessions (i.e. Monday-Friday or Tuesday-Saturday)

It's a Fact!
The following published EMG studies have confirmed that your front and back trunk muscles are coactivated when doing this specific exercise.

✓ **Imai 2010, Ekstrom 2007**

STEP TWO: INCREASE CONCENTRIC AND ECCENTRIC HAMSTRING STRENGTH

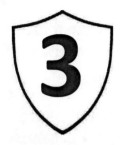

Well that's a mouthful, isn't it? Don't worry, in just a few minutes of reading you're going to know *exactly* what concentric and eccentric strength is – and what it's got to do with bulletproofing your hamstrings...

A Quickie on the In's and Out's of Concentric and Eccentric Strength

Most readers know that your muscles contract to make your arms and legs move around. However not everyone is aware that there are actually *different* kinds of muscle contractions – they're not all the same by any means. In this book, we'll talk about two of them, *concentric* and *eccentric* muscle contractions. Since a picture is worth a thousand words, let me explain by using a couple of them...

Concentric Muscle Contraction

As you lift something, the muscle bunches up and gets *shorter* as it contracts.

Eccentric Muscle Contraction

As you lower something, the muscle gets longer and *lengthens* as it contracts.

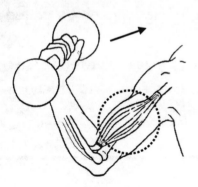

Figure 10.

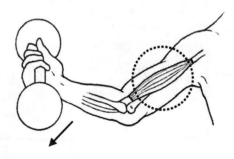

Figure 11.

So as you can see, when a muscle is contracting and getting shorter, we call it a *concentric* contraction. And, when the muscle is contracting and getting longer, we call it an *eccentric* contraction.

Another *super-important* point. Besides the muscle getting shorter and longer, another **huge** difference between concentric and eccentric muscle contractions is *how strong the muscle contractions are.* When scientists have measured the strength of concentric and eccentric contractions, they find that eccentric contractions are *much stronger* than concentric contractions – *which means that your eccentric strength is much greater than your concentric strength.*

To give you a real-life example demonstrating this, if you can lift 50 pounds with one arm (a concentric contraction), you can probably **lower** 100 pounds with the same arm (an eccentric contraction). Interesting, huh? I know this can all be a bit confusing, so here's a quick summary....

Key Differences Between
Concentric and Eccentric Muscle Contractions

✓ When a muscle is contracting and getting shorter, it's called a concentric contraction.

✓ When a muscle is contracting and getting longer, it's called an eccentric contraction.

✓ Eccentric muscle contractions produce much greater force than concentric contractions. Thus, your eccentric strength is greater than your concentric strength.

Well that's all good and fine, but what the heck does this all have to do with your hamstrings?

A lot. For starters, studies show that if you've ever injured your hamstring muscle in the past, there's a good chance that your concentric and eccentric strength is *much lower* than it should be. Consider this study...

- 13 athletes that had a hamstring strain injury in one leg within the last 18 months were compared to a control group of 15 athletes with no prior injury (Opar 2012)

- all athletes were fully active in their chosen sport

- both groups had the concentric and eccentric strength of their hamstring muscles tested

- researchers found that in the group that had strained their hamstrings in the past, the concentric and eccentric hamstring strength in the injured leg was *much weaker* compared to their other uninjured leg

- the control group of uninjured athletes showed no such differences between legs

Hmmm, seems that hamstring strains can often leave you with decreased concentric and eccentric strength! Other researchers have found this to be the case as well...

- this time, 26 athletes with a history of hamstring muscle injury and recurrent strains and discomfort were studied (Croisier 2002)

- the concentric and eccentric strength of the hamstring muscle was tested in both legs at various speeds

- results revealed significantly reduced strength in the hamstring muscle with a history of injury compared to the other leg - for instance, testing found a 10% concentric strength deficit and 24% eccentric strength deficit in the previously injured leg

Weaker hamstrings after an injury? But why? Well, the answer might have to do with the fact that in many cases, parts of the hamstring muscle is frequently found to be *much smaller* after an injury...

- researchers studied 14 athletes who had strained their hamstring muscle 5-23 months earlier (Silder 2008)

- they were compared to 5 healthy control subjects

- everyone had MRI scans taken of both legs

- results showed that 13 of the 14 athletes had injured their biceps femoris (a hamstring muscle) – *parts of which were significantly smaller compared to the healthy controls*

So the moral of the story seems to be that your hamstrings can take quite a beating after an injury. Not only could you lose a lot of your concentric and eccentric strength, but the poor muscle never really gets back to its normal size *in many cases* when scientists look at it on MRI scans.

The good news, however, is that these are problems that *can* be fixed *if* you do the right exercise. The best exercise I know of to solve both of these problems, is an exercise called *the leg curl*. Not only does the leg curl increase concentric and eccentric strength levels, **which can in turn make the hamstring muscle grow bigger**, but it can also help *prevent* hamstring injuries as well. Here's a good example...

- this randomized, controlled trial used 30 soccer players for subjects (Askling 2003). They were divided into two groups of 15.

- both groups followed the same training protocol, EXCEPT one group of 15 players trained on a leg curl machine that involved both concentric and eccentric contractions of the hamstring muscle

- the other group of 15 players, which made up the control group, did not do the leg curl machine

- during the 10-month study period, only 3/15 players in the group that did the leg curl machine injured their hamstrings - compared to 10/15 in the control group!

So if we want to bulletproof our hamstrings, few would disagree that the leg curl is a serious exercise to consider doing!

Three Good Reasons to do the Leg Curl Exercise

✓ can increase concentric and eccentric strength levels which can be significantly decreased after an injury

✓ can make the hamstring muscle bigger – injuries can result in smaller than normal hamstring muscles

✓ can actually help *prevent* hamstring injuries!

The Most Efficient Way to Strength Train Your Hamstrings

Of course the only thing left now, is to show you how to strength train your hamstrings using the leg curl exercise. But before I do that, I'd like to go over some very specific guidelines I want you to use so that you will get the most out of this exercise – in the least amount of time. Because I wrote this book with *everyone* in mind – from the athlete, to the active retired person – it's only wise to make sure that we're all on the same page before going any further.

Then, when we do get down to describing how to do the leg curl exercise, *every* reader will know exactly what I mean when I say, "Do 1 set of 10 reps." So, using a handy question and answer format, let's start with the basics…

How do we make the hamstring muscles stronger?

Muscles get stronger only when we constantly challenge them to do more than they're used to doing. Do the same amount and type of activity over and over again, and your muscles will *never* increase in strength. For example, if Cathy goes to the gym and lifts a ten-pound dumbbell up and down, ten times, workout after workout, week after week, her arms will *not* get any stronger by doing this exercise. Why? Because the human body is very efficient.

You see, right now, Cathy's arm muscles can already do the job she is asking them to do (lift a ten-pound dumbbell ten times). Therefore, why should they bother growing any stronger? I mean after all, stronger, bigger muscles *do* require more calories, nutrition and maintenance from the body. And since they can *already* do everything they're asked to do, increasing in size and demanding more from the rest of the body would only be a waste of resources for no good reason.

It makes perfect sense if you stop and think about it, but we can also use this same line of thinking when it comes to making our muscles bigger and stronger – we simply *give* them a reason to get into better shape. And how do we do that? By simply asking them to do *more* than they're used to doing. Going back to the above example, if Cathy wants make her arm muscles stronger, then she could maybe switch from a ten-pound dumbbell to a *twelve*-pound dumbbell the next time she goes to work out. Whoa! Her arm muscles won't be ready for that at all – they were always used to working with that ten-pound dumbbell. And so, they will have no choice but to get stronger now in order to meet the *new* demand Cathy has placed on them.

For the more scientific-minded readers, physiology textbooks call this *progressive resistance exercise.* You can use this very same strategy to get *any* muscle in your body stronger, and we're certainly going to be using it to get your hamstring muscles as strong as we can!

What's the difference between a repetition and a set?

As we've said, we need to constantly challenge our muscles in order to force them to get stronger, and one good way to do this is to lift a little heavier weight than we're used to using. Of course you won't always be able to lift a heavier and heavier weight *every* time you do an exercise, and so another option you have is to try to lift the same weight *more* times than you did before. As you can see, it's a good idea to keep track of things, just so you know for sure that you're actually making progress – which is where the terms "set" and "repetition" come into play.

If you take a weight and lift it up and down over your head once, you could say that you have just done one repetition or "rep" of that exercise. Likewise, if you take the same weight and lift it up and down a total of ten times over your head, then you could say that you did ten repetitions of that exercise.

A set, on the other hand, is simply a bunch of repetitions done one after the other. Using our above example once again, if you lifted a weight ten times over your head, and then rested, you would have just done one set of ten repetitions. Pretty straightforward isn't it?

Now the last thing you need to know about reps and sets is how we go about writing them down. The most common method used, is to first write the number of sets you did of an exercise, followed by an "x", and then the number of repetitions you did. For example, if you were able to lift a weight over your head ten times and then rested, you would write down 1x10. This means that you did 1 set of 10 repetitions of that particular exercise. Likewise, if the next workout you did 12 repetitions, you would write down 1x12.

What's the best number of sets and repetitions to do
in order to make a muscle stronger?

There was a time when I asked myself that same question. So, in order to find out, I completely searched the published strength training literature starting from the year 1960. I then sorted out just the randomized controlled trials, since these provide the highest form of proof in medicine that something is really effective, and laid them all out on my kitchen table. While getting to that point took me literally months and months of daily reading and hunting down articles, it was really the only way I could come up with an accurate, evidence-based answer.

Now the first conclusion I came to was that it is quite possible for a person to get significantly stronger by doing any one of a *wide* variety of set and repetition combinations. For instance, one study might show that one set of eight to twelve repetitions could make a person stronger compared to a non-exercising control group – but then again so could four sets of thirteen to fifteen reps in another study.

Realizing this, I decided to change my strategy a bit and set my sights on finding *the most efficient* number of sets and repetitions. In other words, how many sets and repetitions could produce the *best* strength gains with the *least* amount of effort? And so, I had two issues to resolve. The first one was, "Are multiple sets of an exercise better than doing just one set?" and the second, "Exactly how many repetitions will produce the best strength gains?"

Anxious to get to the bottom of things, I returned once again to my pile of randomized controlled trials, this time searching for more specific answers. Here's what I found as far as sets are concerned:

✓ there are *many* randomized controlled trials showing that *one* set of an exercise is **just as good** as doing *three* sets of an exercise (Esquivel 2007, Starkey 1996, Reid 1987, Stowers 1983, Silvester 1982). This has been shown to be true in people who have just started weight training, as well in individuals that have been training for some time (Hass 2000).

Wow. With a lot of my patients either having limited time to exercise or just plain hating it altogether, that was really good news. I could now tell them that based on *strong* evidence from *many* randomized controlled trials, all they needed to do was just *one set* of an exercise to get stronger – which would get them every bit as strong as doing three!

And the best number of repetitions to do? Well, that wasn't quite as cut and dried. The first thing I noted from the literature was that different numbers of repetitions have totally different training effects on the muscles. You see, it seems that the lower numbers of repetitions, say three or seven for example, train the muscles more for *strength*. On the other hand, the higher repetition numbers, such as twenty or twenty-five, tend to increase a muscle's *endurance* more than strength (endurance is where a muscle must repeatedly contract over and over for a long period of time, such as when a person continuously moves their arms back and forth while vacuuming a rug for several minutes).

Another way to think about this is to simply imagine the repetition numbers sitting on a line. Repetitions that develop strength sit more toward the far left side of the line, and the number of repetitions that develop mainly endurance lie towards the right. Everything in the middle, therefore, would give you varying mixtures of both strength *and* endurance. The following is an example of this:

The Repetition Continuum

1 rep	10 reps	around 20 reps and higher

strength ⎯⎯⎯⎯⎯⎯⎯⎯⎯⎯⎯⎯⎯⎯⎯endurance ⎯⎯⎯⎯⎯⎯→

Please note, however, that it's not like you won't gain *any* strength at all if you do an exercise for twenty repetitions or more. It's just that you'll gain mainly muscular endurance, and not near as much strength than if you would have done fewer repetitions (such as five or ten).

Okay, so now I knew there was a big difference between the lower repetitions and the higher repetitions. However one last question still stuck in my mind. Among the lower repetitions, are some better than others for gaining strength? For example, can I tell my patients that they will get stronger by doing a set of three or four repetitions as opposed to doing a set of nine or ten?

Well, it turns out that there really is no difference. For example, one randomized controlled trial had groups of exercisers do either three sets of 2-3 repetitions, three sets of 5-6 repetitions, or three sets of 9-10 repetitions (O'Shea 1966). After six weeks of training, everyone improved in strength, *with no significant differences among the three groups.*

And so, with this last piece of information, my lengthy (but highly profitable) investigation had finally come to an end. After scrutinizing *decades* of strength training research, I could now make the following evidence-based conclusions...

> ✓ doing one set of an exercise is just as good as doing three sets of an exercise
>
> ✓ lower repetitions are best for building muscular strength, with no particular lower number being better than the others
>
> ✓ higher repetitions (around 20 or more) are best for building muscular *endurance*

In this book, we'll be taking full advantage of the above information by doing just one set of a strengthening exercise for six to ten repetitions - except for the exercise in the last chapter where we're leaning towards higher reps/holding time in order to boost endurance a little more for improved pelvic stability. So this means that you will use a weight that you can lift *at least* six times in a row, and when you can lift it ten times in good form, it's time to increase the weight a little to keep the progress going. Keeping the repetitions in this range makes sure that we're going to gain more concentric and eccentric muscular *strength*, rather than *endurance*. Lower reps in this range are also very good for increasing muscular size, although the extent to which a person's muscle gets bigger (hypertrophy) from lifting weights is also dependent on other factors as well such as your sex, natural recovery ability, etc.

How many times a week do I have to do a
strengthening exercise in order to get stronger?

Doing the same strengthening exercise every day, or even five days a week, will usually lead to overtraining – which means *no* strength gains. This is because the muscles need time to recover, which typically means at least a day or so in between exercise bouts to rest and rebuild before you stress 'em again. And so, the question then becomes, which is better, one, two or three times a week?

Well, believe it or not, when I went through the strength training literature in search of the optimal number of times a week to do a strengthening exercise, there were a few randomized controlled trials actually showing that doing a strengthening exercise *once* a week was just as good as doing it two or three times a week. However, these studies were done on *very* specific populations (such as the elderly) or *very* specific muscle groups that were worked in a special manner. Therefore, when you take this information, and couple it with the fact that there are a few randomized controlled trials showing that two and three times a week are far better than one time a week, there really isn't much support for the average person to do a strengthening exercise once a week to get stronger. And so, we're again left with another question of which is better, two versus three times a week– which is what much of the strength training research has investigated.

However it is at this point that the waters start to get a little muddy. If you take all the randomized controlled trials comparing two times a week to three times a week, and lay them out on a table, you will get mixed results. In other words, there are some studies showing you that doing an exercise two times a week will get you the *same* results as three times a week, **but** there's also good research showing you that three times a week is *better* than two times a week. So what's one to do?

Well, in a case like this, the bottom line is that you can't really draw a firm conclusion one way or the other. So, you've got to work with what you've got. In this book, we're going to stick with doing the hamstring strengthening exercises *twice* a week. Why do I pick two instead of three?

It's simply a matter of erring on the side of caution – we want to avoid *overtraining* the hamstrings by doing *too* many exercises *too* often. You see, in the next chapter, I'm going to show you a special exercise that heavily works the hamstrings' eccentric strength (very taxing on the muscle). Therefore, since I'm recommending you do *several* hamstring strengthening exercises (one in this chapter, and one in the next chapter), I want to be *very* careful not to overtrain your hamstrings – because then you'll gain little or *no* strength at all!

So this is why you'll be doing hamstring strengthening exercises twice a week - to give your hamstrings plenty of time to rest and recover between workouts. And there's no need to worry that this is not enough exercise either. There is good research showing us that we can get plenty strong working our muscles just twice a week – comprehensive reviews of the literature have confirmed this (Schoenfeld 2016).

How hard should I push it when I do a set?

How hard you push yourself while doing an exercise, also known as *exercise intensity*, is another issue that certainly deserves mention and is a question I am frequently asked by patients. The answer lies in two pieces of information:

1. **Doing an exercise until no further repetitions can be done in good form is called *momentary muscular failure*. Research shows us that getting to momentary muscular failure, or close to it, produces the best strength gains.**

2. **You should not be in pain while exercising.**

Taking the above information into consideration, I feel that a person should keep doing an exercise as long as it isn't painful and until no further repetitions can be done in good form within the repetition scheme.

Does it make any difference how fast you do a repetition?

Many randomized controlled trials have shown that as far as gaining strength is concerned, it does *not* matter whether you do a repetition fast or slow (Berger 1966, Palmieri 1987, Young 1993) – and comprehensive reviews of the literature have reached similar conclusions (Schoenfeld 2015). Here's a look at one of these fascinating studies...

- subjects were randomly divided into three groups (Berger 1966)

- each group did one set of the bench press exercise, which was performed in 25 seconds

- the first group did 4 repetitions in 25 seconds, the second group did 8-10 repetitions in 25 seconds, and the third did 18-20 repetitions in 25 seconds

- at the end of eight weeks, there were no significant differences in the amount of strength gained between any of the groups

So that's the evidence-based guidelines as far as strength is concerned. As far as safety, I recommend that you lift the weight up and down *smoothly* with each repetition, carefully avoiding any jerking motions.

How much weight should I start off with?

For reasons we've discussed earlier in this chapter, I recommend you shoot for doing one set of an exercise for six to ten repetitions. Therefore, you should start out with a weight that allows you to do a minimum of six repetitions, but no more than ten. But how do you figure that out?

Well, by a little trial and error. The first time you do a particular exercise, you're just going to have to take your best guess at to how much weight will allow you to do between 6 and 10 repetitions, try the exercise, and then see how it goes. As an example, say you start the leg curl exercise and decide to try 20 pounds, begin lifting it, and find you can do 8 repetitions in good form. That's great – you've hit our target range of 6 to 10 reps! Next time, you'll use 20 pounds again, and try to do a few more reps, eventually working up to 10 reps before adding more weight.

Now the other thing that commonly happens when you're doing an exercise for the first time, is that you might find that it's either too heavy (maybe you could lift it only once or twice) *or* it's way too light (maybe you could lift it twenty-five times or more). Here again, that's not a big problem. When trying the exercise the next time, simply take another good guess and adjust the weight up or down a little as needed. Do keep in mind that when *anyone* starts a weight-training program, or tries a new exercise for the first time, it's perfectly normal for it to take one or two exercise sessions to find the appropriate weight.

Like I said, it'll be a matter of a little trial and error at first, but do keep in mind that when it comes to strengthening your hamstrings, the main idea is not to see how much weight you can lift, but rather to find a safe starting weight, and then *gradually progress* over time.

And with that last bit of strength-training information, we're finished discussing the basics. So, now that we're all on the same page, let's move on to the leg curl - you only need to do *one* version...

Concentric/Eccentric Hamstring
Strengthening Exercise
~The Prone Leg Curl~

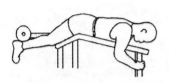 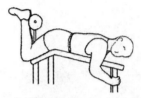 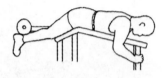

starting position   midpoint   finishing position

Readers who have access to a gym that have weight machines have the option of doing the leg curl exercise on a weight machine. While prone leg curl machines can vary a bit from place to place, they all look very similar to the one in the above picture.

Since it is important that the prone leg curl machine's seat be adjusted appropriately to each individual, it is suggested that the reader consult with knowledgeable staff at their gym facility to help them set the seat correctly.

Doing the exercise is easy. Get into the starting position above, bend both knees to around a 90-degree angle as in the midpoint picture, hold for a second, and then lower both legs down to the starting position – that's one repetition. Doing it this way will increase both concentric AND eccentric hamstring strength!

- ✓ Use a weight that allows you to do at least 6 repetitions. When you can do 10 reps in good form, add some weight.

- ✓ do only one set per day, twice a week, separated by at least one day of rest in between sessions (i.e. Monday-Friday or Tuesday-Saturday).

It's a Fact!
The following published EMG studies have confirmed that your hamstring muscles are highly active when doing this specific exercise.

✓ **Schoenfeld 2015, Andersen 2006**

Concentric/Eccentric Hamstring
Strengthening Exercise
~The Seated Leg Curl~

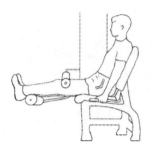
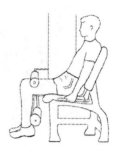
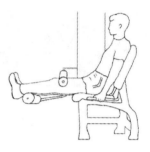

starting position   midpoint   finishing position

Once again, readers who have access to a gym that have weight machines have the option of doing the leg curl exercise on a weight machine. While seated leg curl machines can vary a bit from place to place, they all look very similar to the one in the above picture.

Since it is important that the seated leg curl machine's seat be adjusted appropriately to each individual, it is suggested that the reader consult with knowledgeable staff at their gym facility to help them set the seat correctly.

Doing the exercise is easy. Get into the starting position above, then bend both knees to around a 90-degree angle as in the midpoint picture, hold for a second, and then straighten both legs to the starting position – that's one repetition. Doing it this way will increase both concentric AND eccentric hamstring strength!

- ✓ Use a weight that allows you to do at least 6 repetitions. When you can do 10 reps in good form, add some weight.
- ✓ do only one set per day, twice a week, separated by at least one day of rest in between sessions (i.e. Monday-Friday or Tuesday-Saturday)

It's a Fact!
The following published EMG studies have confirmed that your hamstring muscles are highly active when doing this specific exercise.

✓ **Jakobsen 2014, Ebben 2009**

Concentric/Eccentric Hamstring Strengthening Exercise
~Ankle Weight Options (Pick Only One)~

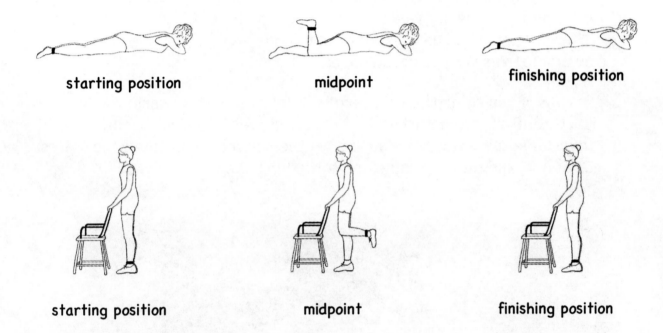

starting position   midpoint   finishing position

starting position   midpoint   finishing position

Readers who do not have access to weight machines can still improve their concentric and eccentric hamstring strength by selecting ONE of the exercises above and using ankle weights.

Either of the above exercises are easy to do. Get into the starting position above, then bend one knee to around a 90-degree angle as in the midpoint picture, hold for a second, and then lower your leg down to the starting position – that's one repetition. Doing it this way will increase BOTH concentric and eccentric hamstring strength!

✓ Use an **ankle weight** that allows you to do at least 6 repetitions. When you can do 10 reps in good form, add some weight.

✓ do only one set per a day, twice a week, separated by at least one day of rest in between sessions (i.e. Monday-Friday or Tuesday-Saturday).

✓ for information of selecting an ankle weight, check out the next page...

A Few Tips on Selecting Ankle Weights

Remember from our discussion on page 22 that muscles get stronger only when we constantly challenge them to do more than they're used to doing. So, this means that taking the same ankle weight, and lifting it over and over again, week after week, simply won't get the job done. Therefore, you'll need to have *several* ankle weights, of varying pounds, available to use as you get stronger.

Now if you think this will involve a lot of money, it certainly doesn't have to. By far, the easiest and cheapest way to go is to buy a set of *adjustable* ankle weights. You can get them at most sporting good stores, or online, and they typically look something like this:

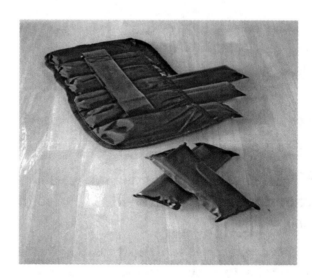

As you can see from the picture, the cuff can attach quite easily to your ankle by means of a velcro strap. Also note that the cuff is made up of six mini weight packs that you can take in and out of their little pockets, depending on how many pounds you want to use. Since the cuff in the picture weighs a total of 10 pounds, and has six little packs, this means that each one weighs a little over a pound and a half. This allows you to increase the weight *gradually* on any given exercise – which is one of the biggest advantages of buying *adjustable* cuff weights.

Some tips on buying them. First, be aware that there are *wrist* cuffs and there are *ankle* cuffs (the above picture shows an ankle cuff). Wrist cuffs are smaller, but I recommend getting the ankle cuffs, mainly because they are heavier which allows you to go up higher in weight over time than the wrist cuffs. Second, pay particular attention to how many total pounds *each cuff* weighs. How much weight should you look for? Probably two 10-pound cuffs will be good to start out with. If the need arises, they do make two 20-pound cuffs, which are also widely available.

As far as cost, I have priced these cuffs at a lot of places and the average cost is around twenty dollars for a pair – not a bad investment considering one pair should last for years with normal use.

So there you have it - four exercises that can increase both the concentric and eccentric strength of your hamstrings. All you need to do now is pick **one** that works best for you (depending on your preference and what equipment you have available) – and then begin!

Noticeable strength gains start after several weeks, with bigger gains becoming apparent after about six weeks of consistent training according to the strength training studies. By doing one of these exercises and "tuning up" your hamstring strength, you'll be taking a giant step towards preventing injury and decreasing any hamstring pain you might have – *the research has proven it!*

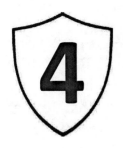

STEP THREE: CHANGE THE STRENGTH CURVE OF YOUR HAMSTRINGS

Since bulletproofing from injury is a major goal of this book, let's take a minute and talk about hamstring strains. This has been well studied, and the research has been able to pinpoint *two* specific types. The first one is...

The High Speed Running Type

This is the most common type of hamstring muscle strain, and happens during, well, high speed running! Interestingly, one part of the hamstring in particular takes quite a beating...

- researchers studied 18 elite sprinters that had first-time hamstring strains (Askling 2007)

- all subjects had MRI's taken of their hamstring muscles after their injury

- ALL of the primary injuries were located in the long head of the biceps femoris

Remember the *biceps femoris* way back on page 10? Here's a quick refresher...

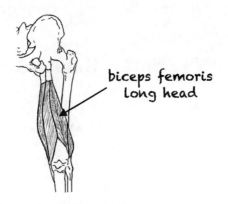

biceps femoris
long head

Figure 12. The long head of the biceps femoris on the back of your *right* leg.

So what exactly happens when you run fast that causes a hamstring strain? Well, it all has to do with *eccentric contractions*. Recall that eccentric muscle contractions produce an awful lot of force in the muscle fibers – much more than concentric muscle contractions. And as you might have guessed, running fast involves *many* of these forceful eccentric contractions over and over. Here's the series of events...

- as you run, you're swinging one of your legs out every time you take a step forward

- of course something has to be able to control the leg swinging forward with each step

- well, it's the hamstring muscle that does this – it contracts *eccentrically* to slow down your leg as its swinging forward

- unfortunately though, these repeated, forceful eccentric contractions of the hamstring muscle can put a lot of stress on the hamstring muscle tissue – and furthermore, the faster you run, the more force (and stress) is created within the hamstring muscle

Looking at it another way, just think of the hamstring muscles as acting as a kind of "brake" to decelerate your leg as it swings forward when you run.

So if you like to run fast, or play a sport where you have to move quickly at times, that *could* be a problem. Question is, is there anything you can do to prevent the most common type of hamstring strain? Absolutely...

The Nordic Hamstring Exercise

The Nordic Hamstring Exercise is one of the most effective tools I have to prevent this type of hamstring strain – and does it work...

- 40 amateur soccer teams were used in this study (van der Horst 2015)

- 20 teams were randomly assigned to do the Nordic Hamstring Exercise, while the other 20 teams made up the control group

- all the teams performed their regular soccer training and were monitored for hamstring injuries that year

- at the end of the study, there were 25 hamstring injuries in the control group, *but only 11 in the group that did the Nordic Hamstring Exercise*

Looks like the Nordic Hamstring Exercise can do a pretty good job cutting down injury rates! There are many such examples in the literature that show this, so without getting too bogged down in research, let's quickly check out one more...

- 50 professional and amateur soccer teams were randomized into one of two groups (Petersen 2011)

- 481 players ended up in the control group and just did their usual training program

- 461 players ended up in the intervention group - in addition to their regular training program, they did the Nordic Hamstring Exercise

- all players were followed for a full soccer season

- at the end of the study, researchers found that the Nordic Hamstring Exercise reduced new hamstring injuries by more than 60%, while recurrent injuries were reduced by 85%

Wow. Not only does the Nordic Hamstring Exercise prevent new hamstring injuries, but it also helps guard against repeated strains as well. But what makes it so effective of an exercise?

Well, it's hard to say with exact certainty, *but* I can tell you several positive things that this exercise does to the hamstrings. The first is that the Nordic Hamstring Exercise *definitely* increases the eccentric strength of your hamstrings – which we learned from the last chapter is crucial in order to bulletproof your hamstrings...

- 18 athletes were randomized to a training group, or to a control group (Iga 2012)

- subjects in the training group did the Nordic Hamstring Exercise for 4 weeks, while the control group did not

- after the 4 weeks, researchers found that the subjects who did the Nordic Hamstring Exercise increased the eccentric strength of their hamstrings up to 21% - while there were no meaningful changes in the control group

The second positive thing the Nordic Hamstring Exercise does, is that *it changes the strength curve of your hamstring muscles to a more advantageous one.* While this may sound really complicated, let me first explain what a strength curve is...

- as you move your arms and legs around, they are actually stronger is some positions than others – this is because the muscles can produce more force at some angles better than others

- a strength curve is just a line that represents these strength changes in different arm or leg positions

- for example, as you bend your arm, the biceps muscle produces its highest force when your arm is at 90 degrees, but not nearly as much as when your arm is all the way straight or all the way bent – therefore, the strength curve of your biceps arm muscle looks like an upside down "U"

If you're a little lost, don't worry, the main thing to be aware of here is that your arm and leg muscles are stronger in some positions than in others - which is represented by a line called a strength curve. So with this knowledge in hand, wouldn't it be nice if you could change the strength curve your hamstring muscles so they could be much stronger in the positions that they get frequently injured in?

Of course! But what position are the hamstrings most susceptible to injury in? Well, with the most common type of hamstring strain, the running type, the hamstring muscle gets injured at the point when you kick your leg out all the way while running. And as I mentioned earlier, the Nordic Hamstring Exercise *can* actually change the strength curve of your hamstring muscle - and make it much stronger in this most vulnerable position...

- 10 subjects took part in this experiment (Brockett 2001)

- all subjects did a single training session of the Nordic Hamstrings Exercise

- researchers measured the strength curve of the hamstring muscle the week before doing the exercise, immediately after doing the exercise, and daily for up to 8 days

- results showed a significant change in the strength curve of the hamstring muscle after doing the Nordic Hamstring Exercise – the hamstrings got stronger in a more straightened knee position

Other experiments have found that the same thing occurs...

- 9 subjects in this study did the Nordic Hamstring Exercise for 4 weeks (Clark 2005)

- hamstring strength was assessed before and after the training

- once again, findings revealed that the hamstring muscle got stronger in a more extended (straightened) knee position

So it looks like we have yet another *fantastic* exercise to help us bulletproof our hamstrings! More good news comes from the fact that you really don't have to spend a lot of time doing it either in order to prevent an injury – a prospective study on professional baseball players found that an average of 3.5 repetitions, per week spread throughout the entire year, was an adequate level to begin to see a therapeutic benefit (Seagrave 2014). On further analysis, the researchers determined that the critical number of repetitions per week needed to avoid injury was >3.5 repetitions per week on average. Nice!

Looks like the only thing left is to show you how to do it...

The Nordic Hamstring Exercise

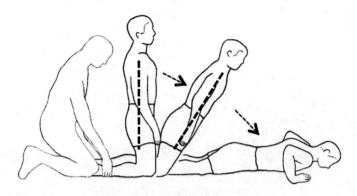

Exercise Movement In Action

The above picture shows the Nordic Hamstring Exercise in action – here's how to do it...

- ✓ kneel on the floor in the above position, getting someone to hold down your ankles

- ✓ as slowly and smoothly as possible, lean forward so that your chest approaches the ground – try to keep your trunk straight

- ✓ put out your arms to catch yourself when you can no longer control your forward momentum

- ✓ allow your chest to touch the ground – then push yourself back up to the starting position - *using your arms as much as possible* - and repeat. You've just done one repetition.

As you can see, the whole point of the exercise is to slowly lower yourself to the ground while keeping your trunk straight - which works BOTH hamstring muscles eccentrically.

How many times (repetitions) is best? Well, no definitive number has emerged yet in the research as being the "magic" number, BUT the research has shown that you have to do at least 4 reps/week to begin to see an injury prevention benefit.

Consider trying a session of 5 reps/twice a week as a starting point, separated by a day or two of rest in between sessions (for example, 5 reps on Monday, and 5 reps on Friday). Work up to that if you have to – your goal being able to control the lowering of your straight trunk 5 times *all the way down to the floor*. To increase difficulty, either add more repetitions OR just try lowering your straight trunk *even slower* to the ground.

And here's another look at one repetition of the exercise...

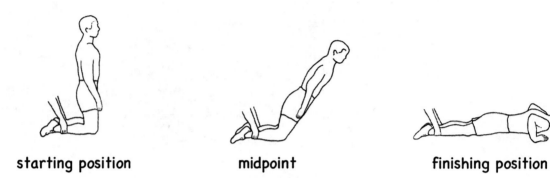

starting position   midpoint   finishing position

A Few Notes

✓ If you don't have anyone to hold down your ankles, it's okay to find something to hook them under - like a couch.

✓ You can put a pillow under your knees – it doesn't affect the exercise

✓ Once again, the goal is to try and lower your straight trunk *all the way to the floor smoothly.* However this takes practice - and most people cannot do this when first starting out. For example, one study reported that subjects could control only the first 30 degrees of downward trunk motion when first doing the exercise!

✓ Exercises such as this one that work the hamstrings eccentrically create a lot of force in the hamstring muscle – so don't be alarmed if you have some soreness in your hamstrings 1-2 days after doing this exercise – that's to be expected.

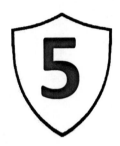

STEP **F**OUR: **M**AXIMIZE **F**LEXIBILITY

Previously, we mentioned that there are two specific types of hamstring strains – each having two *totally* different causes. The first is the "high speed running type" - it is caused by forceful eccentric contractions of the hamstring muscle that take place when one is running at high speeds (such as sprinting).

It is in this chapter, that we now show you how to bulletproof your hamstrings against the *second* most common type of hamstring strain – the "stretching type." As you can probably guess, the cause of this type of strain is when the hamstring muscle is put into a lengthened position - and gets injured by being *overstretched*.

However, unlike the "high speed running type" of strain discussed in the last chapter, this kind seems to take its toll on a slightly *different* part of the hamstring muscle...

- in this study, the subjects were 15 dancers with first-time hamstring strains (Askling 2007)
- each subject was carefully questioned about the details of the injury
- MRI scans were taken on day 2 to 4, day 10, day 21, and day 42 *after* the injury occurred
- researchers found that all the dancers were injured while the hamstring muscle was in a lengthened position
- 87% on the time, the injury involved *the semimembranosus*

Remember the semimembranosus muscle from Chapter 2? Here's a quick refresher...

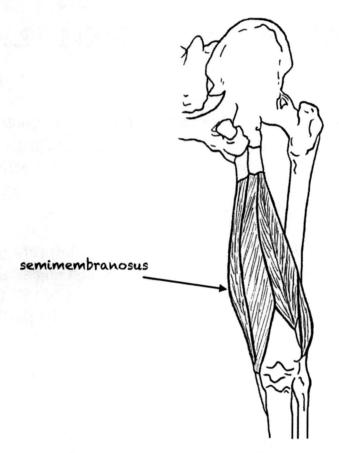

semimembranosus

Figure 13. The part of the hamstring muscle that is most frequently injured when the hamstrings is overstretched – the semimembranosus.

So what can one do to avoid getting this nasty type of hamstring strain? The key, as the title of this chapter tells, is to maximize the flexibility of your hamstring muscle by doing a stretching exercise. This is simply because the more flexible the hamstring muscle is, the less chance you have of overstretching it. Thinking about it another way, the *tighter* your hamstring muscles are, the less stretching they can take, which increases the chances of you getting an overstretch type of strain injury. Of course I can also give you several other *very* good reasons to maximize your hamstring flexibility...

Prior Injuries and Hamstring Flexibility

If you've ever injured your hamstrings, there's a good chance your hamstrings *might* not be as flexible as they should be. Here's why...

- researchers in this study set out to compare the flexibility of injured to noninjured athletes (Worrell 1991)

- the injured group consisted of 16 athletes from a wide variety of sports. All had a non-contact injury of the hamstring muscle within the past 18 months - although they were all currently participating in their sport without any symptoms limiting their performance.

- the noninjured control group also consisted of 16 athletes, but with no history of hamstring injury, matched to the injured group by sport and position

- all athletes had the flexibility of the hamstring muscles assessed

- looking at the injured athletes, researchers found that *the hamstring muscle of the injured leg was significantly less flexible compared to the hamstring of the noninjured leg*

- results also showed that the hamstring injured group was much less flexible compared to the noninjured group

Apparently injuring the hamstring muscle in one of your legs can many times leave it a lot less flexible than the other one over the long run. This highlights the importance of stretching your hamstrings if you've ever injured them in the past - they just might not be as flexible as they need to be!

Stretching = Faster Healing?

Another good reason to stretch your hamstrings comes from a randomized controlled trial done on injured athletes. Let's have a look...

- the subjects in this study were 80 athletes that had just strained their hamstring muscle (Malliaropoulos 2004)

- the first 48 hours, all the athletes were treated with rest, ice, compression, and elevation of the injured extremity

- all athletes were then randomly assigned to one of two groups

- the first group stretched their hamstrings for 30 seconds, repeated four times – once a day. Now the second group also stretched their hamstrings for 30 seconds, repeated four times - except they did this *four times a day.*

- at the end of the study, the group that stretched more frequently (four sessions a day) not only regained their flexibility faster, but also returned to unrestricted activities earlier!

So as you can see from theses studies, the research gives us plenty of good reasons to add stretching to our bulletproof hamstring program.

Benefits of Stretching the Hamstrings

✓ May help prevent "stretching type" hamstring strains
✓ Helps regain flexibility that can be lost after a hamstring injury
✓ Frequent stretching helps speed up healing

Stretching Secrets That Work

While there are many different techniques to choose from when it comes to stretching out a tight muscle and improving knee motions, by far the easiest and least complicated way is known as *the static stretch.* A static (or stationary) stretch takes a tight muscle, puts it in a lengthened position, and keeps it there for a certain period of time. For instance, if you wanted to use the static stretch technique to make your back muscles more flexible, you could simply lie on your back and pull your knees to your chest. Thus, as you are holding this position, the back muscles are being *statically stretched.* There's no bouncing, just a gentle, sustained stretch.

It sounds easy, perhaps a bit *too* easy, so you may be wondering at this point just how effective static stretching really is when it comes to making one more flexible?

Well, a quick review of the stretching research pretty much lays it out straight as there are *multiple* randomized controlled trials clearly in agreement that this is a winning method. Here are the highlights...

- a study published in the journal *Physical Therapy* took 57 subjects and randomly divided them up into four groups (Bandy 1994)

- the first group held their static stretch for a length of 15 seconds, the second group for 30 seconds, and the third for 60. The fourth group (the control group) did not stretch at all.

- all three groups performed *one* stretch a day, five days a week, for six weeks

- results showed that holding a stretch for a period of 30 seconds was just as effective at increasing flexibility as holding one for 60 seconds. Also, holding a stretch for a period of 30 seconds was much more effective than holding one for 15 seconds, or (of course) not stretching at all.

Hmmm. Looks like if you hold a stretch for 15 seconds, it doesn't do much to make you more flexible. On the other hand, holding a stretch for 30 full seconds *does* work – and just as well as 60 seconds!

Wow. So now that we know that 30-seconds seems to be the magic number, makes you wonder if doing *a bunch* of 30-second stretches would be *even better* than doing it one time a day like they did in the study...

- another randomized controlled trial done several years later (Bandy 1997) set out to research not only the optimal length of time to hold a static stretch, *but also the optimal number of times to do it*

- 93 subjects were recruited and randomly placed into one of five groups: 1) perform three 1-minute stretches; 2) perform three 30-second stretches; 3) perform a 1-minute stretch; 4) perform a 30-second stretch; or 5) do no stretching at all (the control group)

- the results? Not so surprising was the fact that all groups that stretched became more flexible than the control group that didn't stretch.

- however what *was* surprising was the finding that among the groups that did stretch, no one group became more flexible than the other!

- in other words, the researchers found that as far as trying to become more flexible, it made no difference whether the stretching time was increased from 30 to 60 seconds, OR when the frequency was changed from doing one stretch a day to doing three stretches a day

So here we have yet *another* randomized controlled trial (the kind of study that provides the highest form of proof in medicine) which is showing us *once again* that holding a stretch for 30 seconds is *just as effective* as holding it for 60 seconds. And to top it all off, doing the 30-second stretch *once* a day is just as good as if you did it three times!

Other randomized controlled trials have also supported the amazing effectiveness of the 30-second stretch done one time a day, five days a week, to make one more flexible (Bandy 1998), and interestingly enough, a later study showed that doing one 30-second stretch once a day, **three times a week** can even make you a little more flexible (Davis 2005) – good to know if you're having a busy week and happen to miss a day or two of stretching!

So as the randomized controlled trials *clearly* point out, it really doesn't take a lot of time to stretch out tight muscles *if* you know how. Based on the current published stretching research, this book recommends the following guidelines for the average person needing to stretch out a tight muscle with the *static stretch technique*:

> • **get into the starting position**
> • **next, begin moving into the stretch position until a *gentle* stretch is felt**
> • **once this position is achieved, hold for a full 30 seconds**
> • **when the 30 seconds is up, *slowly* release the stretch**
> • **do this one time a day, five days a week**

One last note. While it is acceptable to feel a little discomfort while doing a stretch, it is *not* okay to be in pain. Do not force yourself to get into any stretching position, and by all means, skip the stretch entirely if it makes any pain worse.

It Only Takes One Stretch To Get the Job Done

Okay, time for the meat and potatoes of the chapter – the stretching exercise! As the research you've just read shows, all it takes is *one* stretch to make a hamstring muscle significantly more flexible. On the next few pages, you'll find illustrations of how to stretch the hamstrings in *several* different positions. Pick the stretch that is done in the position that is easiest for you – and know that they're both equally effective provided you use the evidence-based stretching guidelines we just covered in this chapter.

Hamstring Stretch #1

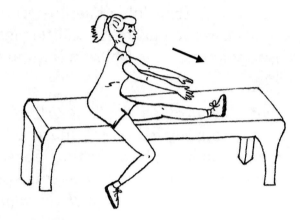

1. Get into the same position as the above picture. It's okay to be on a bed or on the floor.

2. Keeping your back straight, lean forward toward your foot until you feel a gentle stretch on the *back* of your thigh. Try to bend forward from the hips as much as possible, rather than bending from your low back.

3. Try to keep your knee straight.

4. Hold for 30 full seconds.

5. Do this once a day, five days a week. It's okay to work up to the 30 seconds if you have to.

Hamstring Stretch #2

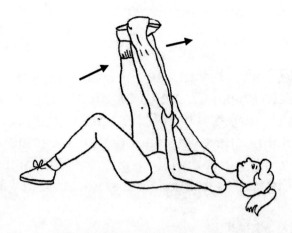

1. Using a towel, get into the above position. It's okay to be on a bed or on the floor.

2. Pull your foot toward you until you feel a gentle stretch in the *back* of your thigh.

3. Try to keep your knee straight.

4. Hold for 30 full seconds.

5. Do this once a day, five days a week. It's okay to work up to the 30 seconds if you have to.

By stretching in this manner, you will be sending a clear signal to your hamstring muscles that they need to elongate. Then, over a period of weeks, the tissues will begin to gradually lengthen bit-by-bit. Also, be aware that these guidelines *are not* for acute (new) hamstring tears/strains – so please consult your medical professional if that's the case.

Pretty simple, huh? If you use the guidelines provided, stretching to lengthen a muscle doesn't have to be an all-day affair. Also, remember to pick only one stretch. Therefore, when stretching both hamstrings, you should be doing one stretch a day per a leg, taking you a grand total of 60-seconds a day to complete – a very minimal investment of your time in an activity that is going to help bulletproof your hamstrings!

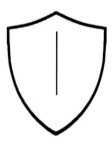

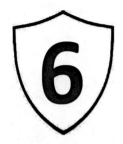

THE BULLETPROOF HAMSTRING PROGRAM

The first chapter of this book explained the idea of *bulletproof hamstrings* – that is, hamstrings that are *pain-free* and *resistant to injury*. It put forth the principle that, hamstring pain is the result of something not functioning properly, and that if the function is restored, the pain will go away. Likewise, improving hamstring function also has the added benefit of making the hamstrings more resistant to injury. Then we addressed the four specific hamstring functions that need to be optimized. As you'll recall, we called them "the four abilities." They are as follows...

- ✓ **A Rock-Solid Base of Support**
- ✓ **Beefed-Up Concentric and Eccentric Strength**
- ✓ **An Optimal Strength Curve**
- ✓ **Maximal Flexibility**

The rest of the book then provided you with the tools you need in order to restore and optimize these four abilities, as well as the scientific rationale for using them. In this chapter, we will put all this information together and put it into action.

The Master Plan

This section will help you organize all of the exercises from the preceeding chapters into an easy and practical program, **THE BULLETPROOF HAMSTRING PROGRAM**. Let's start with an overview of a recommended schedule for you to follow.

DO THESE EXERCISES ON MONDAY and FRIDAY

Exercise to Stabilize the Pelvis (pick one)

The Plank

work up to one minute x 1

Alternative – The Bird Dog

work up to 1 set x 20 reps

Exercise to Strengthen the Hamstrings (pick one)

Prone Leg Curl

1 set x 6-10 reps

Seated Leg Curl

1 set x 6-10 reps

Ankle Weight Option

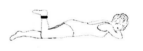

1 set x 6-10 reps

Ankle Weight Option

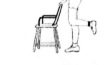

1 set x 6-10 reps

Exercise to Shift Strength Curve of Hamstrings

Nordic Hamstring Exercise

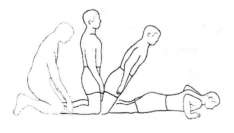

1 set x 5 reps

Exercise to Make Hamstrings More Flexible (pick one)

Hamstrings Stretch #1

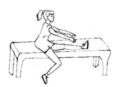

hold for
30 sec. x 1

Hamstrings Stretch #2

hold for
30 sec. x 1

DO THESE EXERCISES ON TUESDAY, WEDNESDAY and THURSDAY

Exercise to Make Hamstrings More Flexible (pick one)

Hamstrings Stretch #1

Hamstrings Stretch #2

hold for
30 sec. x 1

hold for
30 sec. x 1

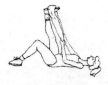

Getting Started

So how exactly do you go about getting started on this plan to bulletproof your hamstrings? Here are a few suggestions...

- First get an okay from your doctor to make sure that the exercises are safe for you to do.

- Next, take a look at the weekly exercise schedule on pages 56 and 57 (the two previous pages).

- Pick a day of the week to start.

- Once you've decided when you'll begin, review the breakdown of exercises for that particular day. If you need more detail on how to do any of them, go back to Chapters 2 through 5 for more extensive instructions.

- On the day you've chosen, jump right in and take your first step toward getting bulletproof hamstrings!

What to Expect

When I give an exercise program to a patient, they usually want to know how long it will take before they start seeing results. The answer lies in how long it takes the body to adapt to the type of exercises I have given. In this book, there are two main types: strengthening exercises, and stretching exercises. As such, there are many published studies showing that your average person can see measurable increases in each of these two areas (strength and flexibility) *in a 6-week time frame.*

Therefore, I would encourage every reader to do **THE BULLETPROOF HAMSTRING PROGRAM** for at least a full 6-weeks to see highly significant gains of strength and flexibility in your hamstrings – as well as a decrease in any hamstring pain you might be experiencing.

Now if you've seen good progress in 6-weeks' time, but you're still not quite where you want to be, continue with the program until you reach your goal. As long as you continue to do the stretches using a thirty-second hold, and increase the resistance of the strengthening exercises as instructed (i.e. adding weight), you should continue to see progress.

On the other hand, if your hamstrings are feeling great after six-weeks, try doing the exercises one time a week for maintenance/prevention, and see how that goes. Make sure that you continue holding the stretches for thirty seconds, and also keep using the same weight you've worked up to for once-a-week maintenance (for instance, if you've worked up to 40 pounds on the leg curl machine, keep using the 40 pounds once a week for maintenance).

A Final Note

The first exercise program I ever wrote for publication was in my book, *The Multifidus Back Pain Solution*. It consisted of three exercises, and I asked the reader to choose only *one*. The exercises were shown to be effective in randomized controlled trials, and if the diligent reader truly followed my specific, evidence-based guidelines, I could all but guarantee that their back pain would improve, if not go away altogether.

Eventually the book was translated into other languages, and as its popularity grew, I started getting some interesting feedback from worldwide readers. Two points consistently came up regarding the exercise routine:

- there weren't enough exercises in the book
- some of the exercises were too simple or they
  were ones that readers had already seen/done before

In case some of these same issues bother you as you reviewed the exercise program in this chapter, I would like to take a moment out to dispel a few common misconceptions before you get started. The first is that some people think you have to spend a lot of time doing a lot of exercises in order to get stronger and pain-free – which is simply untrue. If your exercise program is targeting the *correct* problem with *effective* exercises, then you should not be spending all day doing dozens of exercises. Of course there are exceptions, but they are few.

Another misconception is that simple, uncomplicated exercises are ineffective. Take stretching for example. Leaning forward towards your foot with your back straight, and holding it there for a mere thirty-seconds, once a day, may appear to some readers to be too simple a maneuver, or too short a time frame to ever stretch out a tight muscle. But on the contrary, multiple randomized controlled trials have consistently pointed out that stretching for a longer period of time, or more times a day, will not produce better results.

Finally, the last common misconception deals with not trying an exercise because, "I've done that one before and it didn't help." The interesting thing I've noted is that when you question someone carefully about what they actually did, you often find that while a person may in fact have been doing an exercise correctly, they have *not* been following proper evidence-based guidelines. Using stretching as an example again, let's say that a person tries a particular stretch that is indeed targeting the correct tight muscle, only they've been holding the stretch for fifteen-seconds, instead of the proven thirty-seconds.

After getting poor results for a period of time, most people will usually abandon the exercise and think, "That stretch didn't work." The truth, however, is that they really were doing a helpful exercise - it's just that they weren't following the correct evidence-based guidelines to make the exercise effective.

The moral? When proceeding with **THE BULLETPROOF HAMSTRING PROGRAM**, make sure that you do the exercises *exactly* as instructed, even if you've tried some of them before, or they seem too simple to be effective. Then and only then can you say with certainty that the exercises in this book were really useful or not.

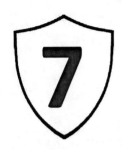

COMPREHENSIVE LIST OF SUPPORTING REFERENCES

It's true! All the information in this book is based on randomized controlled trials and scientific studies that have been published in peer-reviewed journals. Since I know there are readers out there like myself that like to actually check out the information for themselves, I've included the references for *every* study I have cited in this book...

CHAPTER 2

Comfort P, et al. An electromyographical comparison of trunk muscle activity during isometric trunk and dynamic strengthening exercises. *J Strength Cond Res* 2011;25:149-154.

Ekstrom R, et al. Electromyographic analysis of core trunk, hip, and thigh muscles during 9 rehabilitation exercises. *J Orthop Sports Phys Ther* 2007;37:754-762.

Imai A, et al. Trunk muscle activity during lumbar stabilization exercises on both a stable and unstable surface. *J Orthop Sports Phys Ther* 2010;40:369-375.

Kuszewski M, et al. Stability training of the lumbo-pelvo-hip complex influence stiffness of the hamstrings: a preliminary study. *Scand J Med Sci Sports* 2009;19:260-266.

Sherry M, et al. A comparison of 2 rehabilitation programs in the treatment of acute hamstring strains. *J Orthop Sports Phys Ther* 2004;34:116-125.

Snarr R, et al. Electromyographical comparison of plank variations performed with and without instability devices *J Strength Cond Res* 2014;28:3298-3305.

CHAPTER 3

Andersen L, et al. Neuromuscular activation in conventional therapeutic exercises and heavy resistance exercises: implications for rehabilitation. *Physical Therapy* 2006;86:683-697.

Askling C, et al. Hamstring injury occurrence in elite soccer players after preseason strength training with eccentric overload. *Scand J Med Sci Sports* 2003;13:244-250.

Berger R, et. al. Effect of various repetitive rates in weight training on improvements in strength and endurance. *J Assoc Phys Mental Rehabil* 1966;20:205-207.

Croisier J, et al. Hamstring muscle strain recurrence and strength performance disorders. *Am J Sports Med* 2002;30:199-203.

Ebben W. Hamstring activation during lower body resistance training exercises. *Int J Sports Physiology and Performance* 2009;4:84-96.

Esquivel A, et al. High and low volume resistance training and vascular function. *Int J of Sports Med* 2007;28:217-221.

Hass C, et. al. Single versus multiple sets in long-term recreational weightlifters. *Medicine and Science in Sports and Exercise* 2000;32:235-242.

Jakobsen M, et al. Effectiveness of hamstring knee rehabilitation exercise performed in training machine vs. elastic resistance. Electromyography evaluation study. *Am J Phys Med Rehabil* 2014;93:320-327.

Opar D, et al.   Knee flexor strength and biceps femoris electromyographical activity is lower in previously strained hamstrings. *J Electromyography and Kinesiology* 2013;23:696-703.

O'Shea P.   Effects of selected weight training programs on the development of strength and muscle hypertrophy. *Research Quarterly* 1966;37:95-102.

Palmieri G.   Weight training and repetition speed. *Journal of Applied Sport Science Research* 1987;1:36-38.

Reid C, et. al.   Weight training and strength, cardiorespiratory functioning and body composition of men. *Br J Sports Med* 1987;21:40-44.

Schoenfeld B, et al.   Regional differences in muscle activation during hamstrings exercise. *J Strength Cond Res* 2015;29:159-164.

Schoenfeld B, et al.   Effect of repetition duration during resistance training on muscle hypertrophy: a systematic review and meta-analysis. *Sports Med* 2015;45:577-585.

Schoenfeld B, et al. Effects of resistance training frequency on measures of muscle hypertrophy: a systematic review and meta-analysis. *Sports Med* 2016;Apr 21:1-9.

Silder A, et al.   MR observations of long-term musculotendon remodeling following a hamstring strain injury. *Skeletal Radiol* 2008;37:1101-1109.

Silvester L, et. al. The effect of variable resistance and free-weight training programs on strength and vertical jump. *Natl Strength Cond J* 1982;3:30-33.

Starkey D, et. al. Effect of resistance training volume on strength and muscle thickness. *Medicine and Science in Sports and Exercise* 1996;28:1311-1320.

Stowers T, et. al. The short-term effects of three different strength-power training methods. *Natl Strength Cond J* 1983;5:24-27.

Young W, Bilby G. The effect of voluntary effort to influence speed of contraction on strength, muscular power, and hypertrophy development. *J of Strength and Conditioning Research* 1993;7:172-178.

CHAPTER 4

Askling C, et al. Acute first-time hamstring strains during high-speed running. A longitudinal study including clinical and magnetic resonance imaging findings. *Am J Sports Med* 2007;35:197-206.

Brockett C, et al. Human hamstring muscles adapt to eccentric exercise by changing optimum length. *Med Sci Sports Exerc* 2001;33:783-790.

Clark R, et al. The effects of eccentric hamstring strength training on dynamic jumping performance and isokinetic strength parameters: a pilot study on the implications for the prevention of hamstring injuries. *Physical Therapy in Sport* 2005;6:67-73.

Iga J, et al. Nordic hamstrings exercise – engagement characteristics and training responses. *Int J Sports Med* 2012;33:1000-1004.

Petersen J, et al. Preventive effect of eccentric training on acute hamstring injuries in men's soccer. A cluster-randomized controlled trial. *Am J Sports Med* 2011;39:2296-2303.

Seagrave R, et al. Preventive effects of eccentric training on acute hamstring muscle injury in professional baseball. *Orthopaedic Journal of Sports Med* 2014;2:1-7.

Van der Horst N, et al. The preventive effect of the nordic hamstring exercise on hamstring injuries in amateur soccer players. A randomized controlled trial. *Am J Sports Med* 2015;20:1-8.

CHAPTER 5

Askling C, et al. Acute first-time hamstring strains during slow-speed stretching. Clinical, magnetic resonance imaging, and recovery characteristics. *Am J Sports Med* 2007;35:1716-1724.

Bandy W, Irion J. The effect of time on static stretch on the flexibility of the hamstring muscles. *Physical Therapy* 1994;74:845-852.

Bandy W, et. al. The effect of time and frequency of static stretching on flexibility of the hamstring muscles. *Physical Therapy* 1997;77:1090-1096.

Bandy W, et. al. The effect of static stretch and dynamic range of motion training on the flexibility of the hamstring muscles. *Journal of Orthopaedic and Sports Physical Therapy* 1998;27:295-300.

Davis D, et al. The effectiveness of 3 stretching techniques on hamstring flexibility using consistent stretching parameters. *Journal of Strength and Conditioning Research* 2005;19:27-32.

Malliaropoulos N, et al. The role of stretching in rehabilitation of hamstring injuries: 80 athletes follow-up. *Med Sci Sports Exerc 2004;36:756-759.*

Worrell T, et al. Comparison of isokinetic strength and flexibility measures between hamstring injured and noninjured athletes. *J of Orthop and Sports Phys Ther* 1991;13:118-125.

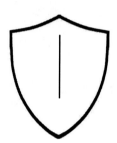

CPSIA information can be obtained
at www.ICGtesting.com
Printed in the USA
LVOW09s1814270318

571329LV00010B/386/P